Intermittent Fasting

TIPS, EATING PATTERN, AND MEALS

My 10 Year Journey of How Intermittent Fasting Changed My Life Making Me Feel Lighter, Healthier, and Full of Energy

by VL DeAlexander

ISBN-13: 978-1-0711-5163-1

CONTENTS

INTRODUCTION

Every man and woman desire to look hot and fit. They want to be attractive and be able to date whoever they like. Not every person can achieve this feat, however. Too many people are struggling with their weight. They're not eating right, and are putting on the fat and calories. Too many people have just let it go and have not taken care of themselves. I realize that I fell into this trap too many times ten years ago when I was but 28-years old, young and single without a wife to take care of. I was a graduate of a liberal arts college with a degree in communications and was drifting through life. Because I didn't have a girlfriend, I wanted to do something more. And later....I found intermittent fasting.

This book is about how I, Victor Lorenzo DeAlexander, became fit with a hot body by doing intermittent fasting and exercise. I am going to introduce each part of my story and include anecdotes and stories that I hope will inspire you to begin a chapter of fasting and exercise. I told you every person wants to look hot and fit, but they don't know how to get there. I think that there is definitely a way to achieve this, but you can't just sit there on your ass and do nothing about it; you have to take action. You have to have a plan. Too much of a person's life is spent in contemplation and complacency and not enough action. People are guilty of not following through with their words, and there are inconsistencies between what they say and what they do.

But you don't want to be that person, I think. You want to be a person of integrity, a person who is true to yourself and wants to accomplish your goals because you are worth it. I believe that every person should be able to reach their objectives if they set realistic, concrete, and achievable goals. That is the only way that they can do it, and I believe that you can also achieve your dreams.

I'm telling my story because it worked. Intermittent fasting changed my life. It made me realize what was important in my life, saved me a boatload of money, and made me feel and look healthier. I also got a hot bod that all the ladies were admiring, and, as a result, I became more confident and happy about my life. It helped me so much, and I believe that you can also do it. I think that you are a person with a purpose. Too many people go through life without a goal, but I believe that you can do it as well. You can get a sexy body because you have a dream to do so. That dream is real and tangible, but you have to believe that it is also something you can reach for and attain. Nothing is impossible. You must understand that all things are possible with a mindset that is positive and growth-oriented.

In this book, I have organized my ideas based on the story that I want to narrate. I show what caused me to go on this journey with intermittent fasting, what worked and what didn't, how I changed my diet and eating patterns, what I did to improve my workout routines, the benefits I have encountered, and the recommendations and tips that I think will help you to build the body of your dreams.

Each chapter is organized with an introduction, life story and lesson, and conclusion, so that you can follow each tip carefully and effectively. I have made this book one that you can reflect on, and it is conversational in nature so that you can pretend that you are in a meeting with me. Imagine we are talking together over a beer or coffee about ways that you can achieve this dream that you have had maybe since you were a boy or girl or teenager. I want you to feel empowered to reach the goal that you've had. It is possible for you to do it. I believe in you. Trust me on this and come with me on this journey. Together, we can achieve what you want. I am offering this book as a means for you to be supported and guided on this journey, based on my own experiences. It will be rough at some points. It was difficult for me, too. I suffered from some severe bouts, but it was all worth it. Like the adage says, "no pain, no gain." You have to take it as it comes. The battle can be fierce and cruel at times, but it is something worth fighting for. There are difficult and great things about this intermittent fasting that I want to share with you, but I also want to show you how to do it and get the results desired.

CHAPTER 1

(YEAR 1)

NOT HEALTHY, NOR ILL ... JUST AVERAGE

In this chapter, I will introduce how I was at the beginning of my journey to better health. I will explain my story in the beginning as an average man looking to improve my health after many essential circumstances.

In the beginning, I, Victor, was just an average guy. There was no ambition in my life. I didn't have a goal that I was going for. Instead, I was just coasting through life, trying to figure out what I wanted to do. Having gone to college, I got my degree in communications. It was a kind of default major that people take just because they want to get a degree. After I graduated, I didn't have a lot of money. I had $30,000 in school debt I had to pay back to my university. When I left school, I could not get a job in my field. I wanted to be a radio host on a radio station in my town. I had, in my mind, an idea to remain in my hometown for the rest of my life. I didn't want to move out on my own, or get my own place. Because I was making less than $20,000 a year working at Starbucks and tutoring on the side, I wasn't able to become financially well-off.

As for my health, I was in pretty good shape. I ate ok. Sometimes, I went out and got drunk and would go clubbing with my friends. I ate at McDonald's frequently, so I gained some weight. Occasionally, I would smoke cigarettes with friends outside. I also went to the Hookah bar sometimes to socialize. The kind of exercise I got was just enough to get by. I went to the gym once or twice a week. I was not maintaining a healthy weight, and had put on a few pounds by snacking every night after dinner.

Although I did some unhealthy things, I could say that I was in average health and didn't have too much going for me. There wasn't too much to comment about it. As I said, I was coasting through my life with no ambition. No desire to get married or settle down. All I wanted to do was stay in my parents' basement and use my hard-earned money from Starbucks to pay my bills and student loans. In that time, I was not happy. I felt trapped by my situation. I wanted to get out of it. I was unsure about how I could proceed. Wasn't there something else I could try for in my life? Why did I always have to eat away my feelings and indulge in little things that were unhealthy? I just thought to myself; it doesn't matter. I'll be this way for a little while, and, eventually, I'll settle down and get married. Right now, I can settle for going out, getting drunk sometimes, going to a club, and working at Starbucks. Later, I can think about going back to school and getting my shit together.

On the surface, you might say I was doing all right. I was just like any average American young man. I didn't have a goal or purpose in life, and indulged in pleasures. That was the way it was with many twenty-somethings out there. Many young people these days are lost. They don't know where to go with their lives. They graduate with so much debt and then can't find a job that will help them repay those loans. I was one of those people. I was among the many people who are struggling to find their way amid this broken system in America. The education system is broken. The job market is broken, and I was one of the people who had to suffer from it.

It was one day when I was 28 that I thought to myself, "What am I doing with my life?" "Why am I stuck in this shithole?" "Why can't I try to get out?" And I realized that I was quite complacent in dealing with the underlying issue of what to do with my life. I was procrastinating. When I lost my mother to breast cancer, I received a wake-up call. I realized that life was painfully short and that I had to do something to live a healthier and more productive life. I had to take inventory of my life and see how I was doing with my health so that I could get a new action plan.

Realizing that life was short and that I had to do something to prolong my life in a good way that does not extend my adolescence, I started looking for a way to do that. I decided to stop procrastinating. I looked up ways to be healthy and read some books about healthy eating and living. I knew I needed an action plan and soon, I would discover what I wanted to do: intermittent fasting.

To conclude, I was able to realize what was important to me. What was important to me was finding a solution to my problem of unhealthy habits. I came up with the answer - to follow a regimen of intermittent fasting that would give me the chance to maintain a healthy weight and to be able to do a lot of great things in my life. Everything is possible, I know that, and I looked forward to seeing what was going to happen.

CHAPTER 2

(YEAR 1)

INTERMITTENT FASTING, WHY NOT?

In this chapter, I will explain how I came up with my decision to give intermittent fasting a try. The media provided me with a source of inspiration, and I was eager to begin this journey into better health, looking good, and feeling great. Here is the story of what happened.

One day, I was on my Netflix binge. Since it was my day off from Starbucks, I was on my computer in my parents' basement, and I had already enjoyed sleeping-in after a long weekend. I then went on YouTube and binged more on videos and things. I did an extensive search of different healthy eating options and ways to live a better life. Suddenly, there was a video that played, and it was Hugh Jackman in X-Men as Wolverine. I saw his amazing body and thought I really wanted to be that guy. He was so ripped and was also quite attractive. Later, I found out how Hugh Jackman was able to get this lean, ripped Wolverine body through a diet from intermittent fasting. Jackman is one of my favorite actors and heroes. I look up to the man. He has been one of my icons. He talked about all the advantages of doing intermittent fasting and how it can benefit your health. And then I thought, "That's it!" "Sweet!" I knew, at that point, that I wanted to do intermittent fasting. I tried to engage in a habit that my hero did, and wanted to be just like him.

That's when I decided that I wanted to do something just for myself to build up my confidence in my body. I knew I had flab and didn't have muscle mass. I tried to look like Wolverine and get big abs and a sexy body that every woman would want. I decided that I really wanted to get healthier and do what Hugh Jackman does. He eats for 8 hours and then fasts for 16 hours. In the YouTube video I watched, he said that most of what a person looks like comes from their diet and what they eat, so I realized that to get buff and fit, I needed to look at my diet and see what I could do to get the physique that I wanted.

To be honest, this was the most ambitious thing that I could try to do. Getting into shape was an essential part of the process because I wanted to take action. I tried to get the body of a sexy dude. I knew that I had to set this goal for myself. It was so important to me. Nothing else had worked for me. I didn't have an action plan for my life. I was still coasting through life, switching my part-time job every year or two but, with this goal, I knew I had something I didn't have before. I was ready for it; I was going to try this intermittent fasting thing.

From the moment of deciding how to do intermittent fasting, I went online and found the different ways people did it and looked at their stories. I became inspired and thought to myself "Why not?" I want to do the same thing. It seems like a great way to get fit and a way to lose the unhealthy lifestyle that I was living in. I then went online and found how you could do this intermittent fasting plan and I started to set some goals for myself, how I wanted to see myself in one month, two months, or in one year. I started charting my feelings and thoughts. It was a fantastic moment for me, and I knew that I could do anything. Perhaps, I would be able to find meaning for my life, because I knew just how important it was to take care of your body.

What is Intermittent Fasting?

In short, it is a way to get your body in shape by not eating for some time. You have an abstemious appetite and can eat adequately for a given time, and then you stop eating and do exercise, and then you go to sleep, wake up, rinse and repeat. You may have reservations about what fasting can do for you because, perhaps, you have heard how hard it is and how you'll get headaches, feel nauseous and not good at times. Well, that's probably going to be the beginning for you. It always sucks in the beginning, but once you get started and get into a routine, it will feel like riding a bike, and you will see and feel the result.

Intermittent fasting has been used by people throughout the world, including Gandhi, Jesus, and other amazing people. You may think it is for the religious and ascetics, but it's not. Anyone can fast. It doesn't always have to have a spiritual component, although, if you're into God, it will help you get close to that transcendent being and will bring you more in-tune with your thoughts and spiritual world. Fasting enables you to be in tune with your spirit and how it works, because, once you stop consuming food, your body is fed not through the physical sensations, but through the elements of the spirit. Your mind is able to focus on the experiences that impact your soul. Intermittent fasting is surprisingly simple and is used by many people around the world. As soon as you have started the routine, you will find that it is so natural that you will think, "How did I not do this before?" It became something that I wanted to do.

Not eating may sound like it's no big deal. After all, living life for saying "no" to the excesses of life seems out of place for this world. Most people love to boast about which restaurant they went to by posting on Instagram, Facebook etc., and showing pictures of their food. But what if there is a simpler way to do it? That's why I decided to do something simpler and more fruitful that could contribute to a lifestyle change. My life needed to be transformed, so I chose the path of least resistance and did something I would say is "minimalistic," in greatly simplifying my life. I have to say, it has made the most significant difference in my life. I am no longer the same man.

In what follows, I am going to show you how this life of intermittent fasting has transformed my life, how it has made me into the man I am today, and how it has led me from being a chubby, no-abs man to a fit and healthy man with a six-pack, who is happy and free. The thing that you have to realize is that you have to set a goal for yourself. You have to set the standard high. No more mediocrity; no more settling for less. You have to own the man or woman that you want to become. You have to hold within your hands the person that you aim to be. You cannot live your life without a goal or objective to go after. Too many people are drifting through their lives, trying to figure out where they should go.

I'm telling you, don't be that person. You have to pursue your passion and do it with zeal. I have learned from this new experience of intermittent fasting that I wanted to achieve an ideal body, diet, and lifestyle. The way to do that was to take the necessary steps and measures. I just had to have a dream and then go after it with all my might. So, what are you waiting for? Let's go on this journey. It is a long journey through my life, but it is a fantastic reflection of how self-discipline, goal-setting, and a bit of hard work and determination have paid off and led me to be a successful man today.

CHAPTER 3

(YEAR 1)

I TRIED EVERYTHING AND HERE'S WHAT I CAME UP WITH

This chapter covers my experience in year 1 when I tried everything to get my weight and diet in order, but nothing was working. I finally tried intermittent fasting and it changed my life. It took some time, but then I sorted it out and decided I would give it a try and that it would change my eating habits. In this chapter, I am going to show you what I did, and then tell you what I'd recommend that you do.

As I was looking for weight management and increasing muscle, I realized I would have to work super hard to get the results I wanted. I tried all the diet plans, including all carb diet, diets filled with protein, and other ones. They always made me feel bloated and not very good. I also tried to take protein powder while I was working out. That didn't work out too well. I was very unhappy with my body type and wanted to seek some help for my situation. I had no idea what to do. The more I worked out, the more weight I was losing because my metabolism was working on overdrive and there was no slowing it down. Also, I tried to eat every 2 hours and then gorged myself with huge meals during lunch to try to get myself to gain weight. I ended up stuffing my face all day, and I felt miserable, had stomach aches, and just felt like crap overall.

My workout routines were not healthy as well. I was running on the treadmill for 2 hours a day and doing cardio like crazy. I was swimming laps four times a week for 1 hour a day. I was also deadlifting four times a week and trying my best to build up muscle while packing my stomach with food. I even took snacks with me to the gym to eat right away once my workout routine had finished. I was racing against time to get myself into shape. It was so freaking difficult. I could never keep up my metabolism with my workouts. It was impossible to do it. I was literally consuming 4,000 calories a day and burning almost all of it because I was exercising so much. And it felt pointless. I was not completing my goals but, then again, I didn't really have any reachable goals. Everything was just put together in a not-so-formal way. I didn't really know what I was doing in this process of trying to buff up. I was not convinced that I could do it.

Looking back at it, I was not doing well. I was trying to manage everything in my own strength and power. I had a poor body image, struggled with who I looked like, and didn't even want to look at myself in the mirror, yet, I aspired to have the body of Arnold Schwarzenegger, or other famous actors with amazing bodies. Knowing that I wanted to get this body and workout, all the same, I wanted to have some options with what I could do, and how I could achieve my goal of that great body that every woman wants to see on a guy.

It was at this point that I decided I had no other option. I needed to do something that would help me to get on track. Intermittent fasting was the option that I chose based on research and looking up different information about how to do it, and I was immediately struck at how easy it was to begin a wellness routine with this method and habit. It just requires you to abstain from food for a period of time. Intermittent fasting allows yourself to take in calories and protein for some time, and work out with the given energy you have. You are then able to see the results of your efforts.

Reflecting on this experience, I realize that millions of people are in this situation. Maybe you are too. You don't know what to do with what you've got. You are unsure how to proceed with your workout routine and diet, so you pack on the protein with shakes, powders and pills. You may also be a person who is working out like crazy and wants to try to add more weight by eating so much to try to increase your metabolic rate. Well, I'm here to tell you, that will not work. It may for a short period, but, after a while, you will either lose that weight which will be burnt off, or you will gain some fat in the process, mainly if you overeat fat or calories. Take heart though, you can achieve your dreams and goals. You should not give up on trying to find the solution. You should not try to do too much or overeat. It is vital that you designate a place for rest and do nothing. Too much workout or food is not going to solve the problems for you. You will need to find ways of relaxing and give yourself breaks from time to time. Additionally, you will have to find a way to use your creativity to live a productive life that is filled with activity and joy. Find an outlet that will help you, whether that is painting, writing, watching films, hanging out with friends, or joining a club.

There is a better way to find the solution to your weight problem, and it is so simple. I tried it, and it worked. Intermittent fasting is going to change your life. Within this method, you will realize that you can seamlessly integrate it into your busy life, and it won't be too difficult. You will be able to accomplish great things by eating only one or two meals a day. You will realize that you can do everything you set your mind to! Nothing is impossible.

When you feel like eating that pizza or burger, go right ahead, because you will be fasting from calories for one or two meals a day. Enjoy! You can find that this routine is going to change and shape the way you eat and work out. No more counting the calories or fat content. You can enjoy a life of freedom and high energy that will make every feat possible.

Conclusion

From what I've told you, I want you to think about giving intermittent fasting a try. You won't be the same person again. You will see the world through a new lens, like never before. If you follow my advice, you will find yourself able to achieve what seemed impossible before. If you do what I tell you to do, you will be able to lose those pounds that you put on because you didn't eat right. Also, you will be able to get that hot body that you always wanted, and you will be super fit because you can follow a workout routine that will help you to build muscle mass.

I'm Victor, your guide on this journey. I've been there, done that. You can trust me because I have seen and done it all. Throughout my 10-year voyage, I saw a lot of development in my own body and workout routine, and I believe that you will also see amazing results. I want to be here to support you through your time. I tried it all and then came to this point where I could do nothing else. Allow me to guide you through this thing. We can do it all together. Don't be afraid or anxious. This journey is meant to be done with someone else. Let me and a friend or buddy help you to achieve your goal. All things will happen at the right time. I'll cheer you on the whole way.

CHAPTER 4

BENEFITS OF INTERMITTENT FASTING

Now that you have chosen to give intermittent fasting a try, I want to educate you about the benefits of intermittent fasting that have been proven by research. In this chapter, I will highlight the types of things that you can get out of pursuing this life of wellness. Here are some things to bear in mind as you are feeling more motivated to do this thing.

You may be wondering, why not eat whenever I want? Why shouldn't I just eat as much as I want of healthy food sources? In my opinion, if you give your whole system a break from food and give your stomach some rest time, you will see a wide range of benefits that I want you to see for yourself:

• Lowers the risk of cancer. One study has proven that when you modify the frequency and timing of eating, you can influence the use of insulin and decrease the risk for breast cancer in women.

• Helps you have a healthy heart. Intermittent fasting can lower your risk of heart disease because your triglycerides and blood pressure are reduced and it also gives you healthy cholesterol. I went to the cardiologist for a test last year, and I was able to find out that my heart was healthy, as if it were 25! That means that this intermittent fasting is doing something for me.

• Helps you to lose weight quickly. Intermittent fasting is going to help you to lose weight faster as you can lessen leptin resistance, which causes your body to store fat for energy instead of burning it (William Cole). While I didn't have a problem directly with this, I was able to successfully manage my weight over time after doing intermittent fasting as I've mentioned above.

• Allows you to stop craving so much food during the day. When you do intermittent fasting, you will stop craving food when you're hungry. I'll be honest about this one. I used to snack all the time and gained some fat on my belly as a result. I was not a happy camper. Once I started intermittent fasting, I realized that I could go for stretches of time without snacking. It was amazing!

• Helps to improve your lungs. Another study has shown that intermittent fasting can decrease symptoms of asthma, as well as stress (William Cole). For this one, I was able to improve my lungs over time. I had my full body scan, and the doctor said my lungs were super healthy. I was delighted to hear that point.

Intermittent fasting helps you with your overall energy levels. When you store energy from your food, you're able to release it when you're active again. Usually, this will entail working out during the period when you eat, and then resting during fasting periods. You will notice a tangible difference in your energy level and feel more hyper and energetic as a result of these fasts.

You will feel happier and more productive. I felt the difference and was sincerely happy when I first started this type of fasting. It made me feel like I was "on top of the world" and I could do anything I wanted. There is a seriously empowering feeling that you experience whenever you are doing this intermittent fasting routine.

You will struggle less with depression and anxiety. When you eat healthily and do the right kind of exercise, you will find that you can get less anxious or depressed. A lot of what we eat determines what our moods will be like, so the best thing is to stick to a plan that will strengthen our immune system and help us to feel better. I was able to enjoy my food and have a period of no eating. It helped me to feel secure and it stabled my moods because the fat was being stored in my body over time. It was great.

These are some of the benefits I have been able to find out while researching and pondering. There are a host of others that I was able to discover, but I wanted to inform you about what I was able to find. Intermittent fasting will be a type of program you want to be on, not just for the short-term, but for the long-term, as well. It is going to help you achieve long-term health benefits because you're willing to submit to a disciplined program that will work wonders for your lungs, gut, and heart. I'm telling you it is worth it!

I know I had some difficulties motivating myself to do this. I didn't want to have to skip a meal a day and go for periods where I would be hungry. Believe me, it can feel like a huge sacrifice that you're making every time you do this but, after I read about the benefits, I felt more motivated to keep going with it. Research has extensively proven the effectiveness of intermittent fasting, and that's where I knew that I was doing the right thing. If many scientists were proving how great it was, then I knew that it was going to be something that would work wonders in my life.

So, what are you waiting for? Don't you believe in the power of science and research? They support the decisions I make in my life. You also have to follow what research is saying because, often, these studies are proving the point that you should do something to improve your overall health, and the majority of studies have shown the positive aspects of intermittent fasting. No wonder so many people are getting into it today. They see how intermittent fasting helps them get into shape, benefits their immune system, and gives them a sense of purpose and meaning to their lives. People know that this type of fasting is going to help them get their health on the right track. No more worrying about what goes into their stomach or uselessly counting of all the sugar and fats that a person is taking in. That's nonsense. Don't waste your time on the things that are not effective. Do things that are proven to work. Intermittent fasting is going to help you do just that.

Conclusion

To conclude, as I was thinking about intermittent fasting, I realized that science was proving just how great it was. I am a believer in the progress of humanity and that, through scientific achievements, we can make the world a better place. Having examined the research that has been conducted on this topic, I knew that I wanted to educate people on how wonderful intermittent fasting could be. I hope that you will see how you can also benefit from it.

CHAPTER 5

(YEAR 2)

THE OBSTACLES: PAIN AND STRUGGLE

In this chapter, I am going to be frank and candid about the struggles and pain that went into intermittent fasting during my second year. I will share my insights on how I handled these situations and then I will go into tips for coping with the challenges that you will inevitably face. I am also going to offer you some solutions.

When I first started fasting, it was a hard time for me. I felt anxious the first few days I was trying to fast because I was scared of not eating at my regular times. I was also afraid of losing muscle mass because I was not eating. I thought I would lose more weight than gain any, so I was quite skeptical about it. Also, I felt ashamed that I was trying this method because I thought my parents would not approve and that they would make fun of me for trying to do this fasting. I also thought that people would not understand and think I was starving myself. I would get criticism from everyone I met because they would say to me, "Victor, you're so skinny. You shouldn't be starving yourself. You have to feed yourself with something. Eat a burger from Burger King. Do something to up your fat and calories." That would make me feel ashamed and embarrassed.

In the past, I had told my friends and family that I wanted to become a pescatarian or a vegan. Within a few weeks, I quit doing it, because they said to me I need to eat more meat and carbs. I listened to them; therefore, I felt cautious about giving people information that I was going to start fasting.

As for my physique, I had a lot of fat on my body. Although I was lean, I struggled with strength training. I was overeating and cultivating some seriously bad habits. Unfortunately, those bad habits caused me a lot of heartaches as I was starting the plan. I began the program with many mistakes that I want to share with you. They were difficult, and I learned from them, but they caused me a great deal of pain.

Mistake #1: Not Keeping the Time

The first mistake I made in doing this plan was not watching the clock. Basically, I would eat whenever I felt hungry. In the beginning, I didn't have set meal times and would just eat anytime but, as I started the intermittent fasting, I realized that I had to have set meal times that I could sit down and have my meal. I realized that I had to program myself so that I could do that, but I was so lazy and only wanted to feel satisfied. As a result, I got off to a rough start and didn't lose any weight during my second year.

Mistake #2: Lack of Hydration

The second mistake I made was not being hydrated through the day. As a result, I got these intense headaches that were horrible. I even had to go into hospital for not hydrating my body correctly. It hurt like crap. I was so miserable. At that hospital visit, I thought I was going to die, both of thirst and hunger. The doctor had to plug up an IV to me to keep me hydrated. Never again.

Mistake #3: No Accountability

The third mistake I made was not having someone to keep me accountable. Every person needs a trusted friend to help them to make it through. No accountability = no progress. I felt that I needed to have someone to check in with me throughout this process, but I was stubborn and thought, "Oh, ok, I'm fine. I'll just deal with it all on my own."

Mistake #4: Drinking My Coffee with Cream and Sugar

For a while, I thought I could deal with the problem of hunger by drinking more coffee, and that would help me make it through; then I started cheating on my calories. I started adding milk or cream and sugar to my coffee to make it just like a meal and, when I did that, I inadvertently stopped my fast. This was something that I shouldn't have done, but I was doing it, all the same. Now I realize it was dishonest and I shouldn't have done it. If you're drinking coffee, drink it straight black with no added ingredients.

Mistake #5: Eating Too Much of the Wrong Kinds of Food

I started out with this chapter talking about how I ate a lot of junk food. I would eat pizza, burgers, chips, among other kinds of junk food, all because they would fill me up and I would feel satisfied in the end. When I became 30-years old, I realized I had to get better at my eating habits. I needed to eat foods that not only were going to satisfy me and fill my stomach, but also benefit my health. I had to change from filling up on so many high-calorie foods, so I had to make some changes to my diet.

Mistake #6: Doing Too Much Activity While Fasting

When I started with intermittent fasting, I did too much heavy lifting and exercised in my fasting period, and I began to lose some muscle from all that training. I checked my weight after a few times of fasting and exercise, and I would lose 3-5 pounds at a time. Because I am lean, I could lose weight super quick, so keeping on weight was quite the challenge for me. Having too much workout and activity caused me to lose weight and muscle, which was not helpful for me, as I wanted to get a healthier body type and a fit physique like the Wolverine.

During the period of the first two years, I was struggling to get into a routine of fasting. I tried different things, got too ambitious, wanted to find some ways of coping with hunger pain and other things, and ended up having some unfortunate experiences. I had to learn a lot about how to do the intermittent fasting based on the different available plans. I wanted to quit. I'm not going to lie. It sucked sometimes. I was struggling to have a reason to keep going, and I also ended up having some depression and mental health issues, as well. I realized that it was hard for me and I needed someone to support me through this time.

My Recommendations for You

What I recommend you do is not making the same mistakes that I made. First of all, don't go in without planning how you're going to do your fast, or how long you will do it for. Plan for failure. You have to go in with a plan, knowing exactly how you're going to execute it. Secondly, you will need to drink a lot of water during your fast. Because your body is burning calories while you're fasting, you will need to replenish its supply of water. Don't make the mistake of having to go into hospital like me and have an IV connected to you. It's just not worth it. Thirdly, drink your coffee black. Don't add anything to it. Don't try to cheat your way to fasting. It's not honest, and it's lying to yourself and others. You have to be a person of integrity, and the only way that you'll get ahead with this is by following the guidelines of fasting. Fourthly, find someone you know who you can tell about your plan to fast. Allow that trusted friend to be your accountability partner. Talk to that person and tell them when you're fasting, so that they can be a supportive person. Fifthly, you should talk to your doctor about your plan. Let them know that you're planning on doing intermittent fasting. It's crucial that they understand what you're going to do so they can make health recommendations that you should listen to. Next, you have to eat the right kinds of foods. In the sixth chapter, I will go into what types of foods you definitely should eat. You don't want to fall into the trap of eating the wrong kinds of foods because that will not help you achieve your weight-management goals. Finally, exercise in a reasonable frame of time with good intensity. You want to do your best, but don't overdo it, because that will be counterproductive and will not enable you to finish what you start. Fit in a workout plan that will help you eat during a designated period. Also, you should find a time to rest your body from all the working out that you might be doing. It's vital that your body finds times to rest from all the energy that it is exerting.

Conclusion

As you can see, there are certain things that you should avoid in your intermittent fasting plan. You don't want to be without a plan at all. You have to be specific with your goals and stick to your project. Don't deviate from what you have written down as your plan. You also have to be careful to watch out for all the health concerns that there might be. Without the proper consultation with a physician, you might be in for trouble, so talk to your doctor before you start a plan. Finally, maintain a healthy balance with exercise, diet, and rest, and you will be on your way to a successful routine that could change your life.

CHAPTER 6

(YEAR 3)

COOKING MY OWN MEALS

This chapter discusses one strategy that I used to become healthier - cooking my own meals. I will give you some of the tips and strategies that I used to make this part of my wellness routine work.

When I first started thinking about how I would do this intermittent fasting thing, I realized that I wanted to make myself healthier, so I stopped going to McDonald's and eating fried foods all the time. I then discovered that I actually liked to cook. I guess I only needed to give it some time; enough time for me to make a delicious recipe or something that I would like that's also super healthy. In the following paragraphs, I will explain how cooking my own meals transformed my way of thinking and led me to a new chapter in my life.

First, once I got the diabetes diagnosis, I knew that I needed to take inventory over my fat and sugar intake. It was getting way out of control. I was eating too many fried foods and drinking fizzy drinks. It was getting out of hand. I was also spending too much on food every month. There was just too much. Too much on the portion sizes. Too much on the cost. I lived for excess. I finally had an epiphany in which I realized I needed to eat more healthily or else I would become obese; therefore, I decided to cook my own meals — the best decision I could make.

As a single man living alone, I wanted to figure out how to cook the best and most delicious meals that I could make. I watched Food Network and Martha Stewart Living for more information. Don't laugh at me. Those are good shows, even for men looking to up their game in the kitchen. Instead of spending a lot of money on drinks and going out with friends, I ended up spending the money on organic food with fruits and vegetables from different stores, such as Greenlife. It was the best investment for me, and I ended up saving around $200 each month on all that food. It was great. Furthermore, that money could go back into the debt payments that I needed to make every month. It worked out well with my finances.

How Cooking at Home Helped Me

Cooking at home was a great thing because I didn't look to be going out all the time to eat any longer. I could stay in and make amazing fancy meals for one. I could also focus on what was the most important thing for me - enjoying life and being a "live-to-eat" person, rather than an "eat-to-leave" type. I also started to slow down as I ate my meals. I truly enjoyed the opportunity to indulge in every bite of my Fettuccine Alfredo, courtesy of Giada De Laurentiis. It was amazing to discover all the best recipes on the Food Network and apply them to my kitchen and, at the age of 30, I started to invest in the cookware that would make me enjoy working in my kitchen. It was fantastic. Cooking at home was also the answer to my weight-management plan. I was able to eat well and not spend too much money. I had to come up with ways to make things better for myself, so I resorted to cooking my meals, and it made a huge difference.

What Types of Things Did I Cook?

As I got more creative with cooking, I realized that there is not much you have to do to get the results that you want. All you have to do is use the same essential ingredients and then you can do almost anything with those ingredients. I started with making eggs, bacon, and biscuits, which would give me a high carb and protein diet. I realized that I needed to cook more of protein and carbs because I had low muscle mass and was a very skinny person. I had very little in the way of muscles. Because I had eaten just any way I wanted before, I was struggling to get rid of my fat that was on my belly. I also wanted to gain more weight, but also increase muscle mass. I started cooking meals such as pasta carbonara that had cheese, egg, and bacon. This helped me to develop a repertoire of healthy and filling meals, but it wasn't just the carbohydrates that I added to my diet. I also made salads - green salads. I developed a desire to make my balsamic vinaigrette and added feta cheese, mushrooms, tomatoes, and green peppers to make a delicious meal. I then added a few slices of toast with avocado spread to the mix. It was amazing. I made so many simple meals that I was able to enjoy daily, and I didn't feel the temptation to go out and splurge on that meal at a restaurant. Going out can easily cost a fortune from $20 - 25 in a regular restaurant, and I didn't want to break the bank anymore. It was too much for me.

What Was My Budget for the Food?

Before starting this routine of cooking my meals, I was easily blowing over $500 on food and drink. Every night I was going to a restaurant with friends or having a glass of wine with my meals. I was doing so much work that I had no desire to go home and prepare my lunch because I was so exhausted from the job. Many times I would order delivery at $30 a pop for pizza and wine or beer. I was entirely frivolous with my expenses and did not watch what I was spending and ended up with very little money at the end of the month. Unfortunately, I was careless. After starting this new routine, I noticed I was a lot more careful with my expenses and looked at my wallet and made the right decisions, especially when it came to grocery shopping. I have no regrets. It was a great thing to do, and I am thankful it all worked out the way it did.

My Recommendations for You on this Adventure

As I consider what is essential, I believe that making your own meals at home is very productive and also healthy. If you go to a restaurant, you never know how many hands have been touching that burger or fry that you order. Also, it is quite uncomfortable to be in a restaurant eating all the time, where there are a lot of germs, not to mention the fact that so many additives are put on the food that makes it quite unhealthy. This is why I am all for the idea of finding ways to prepare food at home. It's not hard.

The main thing you need to do is to master the basics of cooking at home. You have to find a few ingredients and make the same meal over and over with those ingredients. Go online and search for ways you can spice it up by adding ingredients or using a different recipe. Consult Food Network or Martha Stewart. You can always find some creative ways to spice up that PB&J or grilled cheese. There are so many recipes out there you can try. All you have to do is go online, and you will find the solutions there. Find the best ingredients you can. You can order your food online, or go to the store and pick everything out on your own. It is essential to find the right ingredients that will be healthy with no additives and no MSGs. This is crucial to giving you a healthy diet.

Why Your Diet is Important

In addition to the tips about cooking at home, you should know just how important it is to keep your diet under control. If you want to buff up or develop a better body, you will have to watch what you eat. You should eat lots of protein, carbs, fruit and vegetables. A balanced diet is so vital to giving you the result that you desire. The only way you're going to get fit is by focusing mostly on your diet because that will influence how you get more muscle mass. I realized I wasn't eating right and that was why, no matter how much I went to the gym, I was still not getting the results that I wanted in my muscles; therefore, I recommend focusing on how you can make your diet the best that it can be.

Conclusion

My conclusion is that diet and making your meals at home will give you a wellness routine like no other. You have to learn to slow down. This world is too fast-paced. We go through the drive-thru at McDonald's when we feel like it. Too much of the food we consume is fast food and full of MSGs and additives that are quite toxic and can cause sickness or worse. I had a crisis of discovering I had diabetes that made me watch what I ate and helped me to take control of the fat and other things I consumed. Don't wait until it's too late to find a solution to this problem. Act now. Your health is so important. Take good care of yourself.

CHAPTER 7

DIET PLANS FOR INTERMITTENT FASTING

In this chapter, I will talk in detail about how I started to develop the diet plans that would help me as I did my intermittent fasting. I will talk about my story, and then I will offer you some recommendations for what you can do to get the most out of your diet plan.

During my third year, I had started developing my meals at home. This was the first time that I had gotten my own place, so I was super excited. Armed with the knowledge that I had about intermittent fasting, I wanted to cook some super simple meals at home.

I'm now going to talk about some diet plans that worked for me and helped me to manage my weight and energy levels all the time. I will start out with the program that helped me the most in the beginning. I did some research on this matter, so I could get it right. I will show you what I did at each step of the process, so you can get an idea of what you can do for your diet plan.

When you start your intermittent fasting journey, you will probably see that you feel fuller for a more extended period, and that you will be able to eat more naturally. In the following plans, I will show you what I did for each part of it, and how I fitted in the meal times around my fasting schedule.

1.   The 8-6 Meal Plan

Here is an example of what I did for a while at the beginning of my fasting. I would eat between the hours of 8am and 6pm. I was able to find the right balance with fasting and eating and get a taste of what it was like to fast. It was still a 14-hour fast, and it was instrumental in helping me to improve my metabolism. Let me show you what I ate during that time.

Breakfast: Avocado   smoothie   with blueberries at 8am

In the morning, I would begin my day with a protein-packed smoothie that was easier to digest having fasted the night before. Often, I would get sick when eating breakfast in the morning because I would feel woozy and not very good. In the beginning, I started by binging on pancakes, biscuits, bacon and eggs. I realized that this was not healthy and that I was killing my weight plan goals, so I soon resorted to smoothies in the morning, which helped me to get going before I would have lunch at noon. The ingredients of my smoothie would include protein powder, avocado, kale, chia seeds, blueberries, and coconut milk. Basically, I would grab all of these ingredients, put them in the blender, and go to town with it. It felt great, and I soon realized that I was eating healthier and having a higher level of energy. It did wonders for my health.

Lunch: Veggie burgers at 12:30pm

During the week, I went to Greenlife grocery and would get veggie burgers, which are packed with energy. They are simple, but effective to cook at home. In addition to the veggie burger, I would put leafy lettuce on top of them, garlic powder, and cumin to top it off. It was always delicious and easy to prepare. I would cook them on the stove top at home and put them on a bun. It was a great way to cook and have a good meal at home.

Snack: Cinnamon rolls at 3pm

I didn't have to skimp on sugar intake during this time, so I would give myself a meal around 3pm, and it was terrific. I was able to provide myself with some sugar and fat right before dinner. Cinnamon rolls are quite delicious and also easy to prepare. You just have to give yourself the time to do it during the day.

Dinner: Tuna and veggies at 6pm

Fish can be a great way to get your omega-3 fats in your diet. I love to eat tuna salad from time to time. You can also make this into a sandwich, which is particularly delicious. For example, you can go to the bakery and get a baguette slice or something and then add it to this mix. Then, you can stir fry some vegetables. Add yogurt or a cookie for dessert, and you have a great meal at the end of your day, which is high in nutrients.

This plan worked for me for a couple of years. I was struggling to find a way to eat at designated times, so, when I tried this plan, I was able to schedule my eating between this window, and it helped me to achieve even better results. This plan can be used for beginners, who are just starting with their fasting routines. As I went along, I wanted to challenge myself to fast for more extended periods, and it was at that point that I was able to make even more progress with my wellness plan. As I went with the 8-6 program, I started to notice how my appetite would get more abstemious, and I no longer felt too hungry or had a stomach rumbling throughout my day.

2. The 12-6 Meal Plan

The next step I took was the 12-6 meal plan in my third through fifth years. I was able to make some significant progress in my weight-management during this time, and I felt a lot more energetic. In this plan, you have the same structure of an 8-6 meal plan, but you add an extra 4 hours to your fasting. During my work week, I would do this fasting routine. Instead of eating breakfast, I would drink 2 cups of coffee to start the morning. With this plan, I would be eating between the hours of 12pm and 6pm, with a full 18 hours of fasting during a period of 24 hours.

Although I was skipping breakfast, I knew that I needed to still drink a ton of water. The first time I tried this method, I failed to give myself enough water or fluids, and I had a terrible cramp and headache during the fast. It was rough. I also had to take some herbal tea to make me feel even more hydrated during my day. Because I had increased my fasting period, I needed to add even more fats to my diet; therefore, because I had a burger during that 8-6 window, I was able to add even more energy to my plan. It was amazing. Besides, I also saw myself adding more fruits and snacks that were high in fat content to be consumed around 3pm. Around dinner time at 6pm, I kept on with the meal plan that I did before with the 8-6, but then I would fast for an even more extended period.

The 12-6 plan was going to help me achieve my weight loss goals. I gained a little bit of fat on my bones over the years and had some problem with my muscle mass but, once I started this plan, I noticed that I was able to burn more fat and then that flab that I had on my belly was disappearing, and I knew that it was doing me good.

3. The 2-day Plan

Then, around year 5, I wanted to change everything up and wanted to modify my fasting. I knew that I wanted to take a rest from all the fasting and eat just a little bit on certain days. I also had lost weight over time and needed to keep on some pounds, as I was trying to gain muscle mass. So, what I did was do a modified plan, where I would eat anything I wanted to on five days, and then, for two days, I would only eat about 500 calories for those days. On the days where I wasn't fasting, I had to make sure I was getting enough fats, protein, fruits, and vegetables, among other things, to get my daily intake of essential nutrients. On the fasting days, I chose to eat smaller meals or snacks throughout the day, and then I would eat only some meat and cheese without bread for those days. I used some health and wellness apps to make sure I didn't go over 500 with the caloric intake.

This plan made it a little tougher for me. I started to have cramps and would get headaches because I was eating so little on a few days of my week. Then, I would binge on calories, fat, and carbs on my non-fasting days. It ended up being a bit complicated, and I was not happy with the overall result. This plan was harder to get right, so I wouldn't recommend it, except for the more advanced person to do, because it is going to be quite difficult some days. You should also consult a doctor before trying this kind of plan because it can be hard on your system. If you are taking medication, then it could be dangerous to engage in this type of fasting; therefore, you should exercise caution when trying out this way of fasting.

4. The 5-2 Plan

In this plan, I decided that I would eat for five days and do no eating for two days that are not in a row. For example, I would fast on Monday and Wednesday, but eat as usual on the other days of the week. On the five days, I would eat the same kinds of foods as before, including high-fat content, protein from meats, and fruits and veggies. I tried out this routine when I was in about years 6 and 7, and it was effective, but I would get hungry a lot more easily, as I think my body was burning at a faster rate. Combine this with an intensive workout, and you get a result that is losing weight and muscle mass; therefore, I would only recommend this fasting to someone who is well into their fasting routine after a few years of having done it. The method of fasting is not for beginners and can cause health problems if you are not careful. Please exercise caution with this one, as well.

5. Every-other-day Plan

This method of fasting proved to be one that provided breakthroughs in my life. I only resorted to it after the first seven years of doing fasting. It allowed me to build muscle power and stamina. My workouts were much better. I got sore less throughout the week, and I was able to recover from my workouts, as well. It helped so much. I also saw that I was ready to go for more extended periods without eating. I don't recommend this type of plan for beginners. You're going to have to wait a long time before you have the stamina for this plan because you will have to go for days without food throughout the week. You alternate the days that you fast, but you should still fill your diet with good meat and protein sources, good fats, fruits, and veggies. On the fasting days, you should drink lots of water and herbal tea, as well as some coffee and black tea. I would say that this one helped me a lot. If you're an experienced faster and you want to go the distance with your fasting, try this one out, but make sure you're getting the right foods into your system because you don't want to faint on the side of the street due to exhaustion. Proceed with caution.

The Warrior Diet

The final step in my journey to achieving the right balance with my dieting was the Warrior Diet. It is a type of intermittent fasting that includes a reduction of caloric intake for a period of time. It is based on the concept of warriors who ate very little during the day while they were on the hunt for food, and then they feasted for dinner. Ori Hofmekler founded it in 2001. In this plan, you fast for 20 hours a day and then eat as much food as you want at night; however, during the 20-hour window, you should consume a small amount of dairy, including eggs, fruits, and veggies, as well as plenty of fluids, including coffee, tea, and water. Following this period, you can eat as much food as you want from any type within 4 hours; however, you shouldn't eat too many processed foods during that time.

To get started with this plan, I followed a rigid three-week plan that allowed me to get to the point where I wanted to be. I will write later about that in this chapter. When I did this plan, I burned lots of fat, was able to concentrate on my work, and got spikes of energy that were just too good. It was terrific, and I felt a huge difference. It was like I was on top of the world.

Now, because this plan is so extreme, there was no way I could keep doing it for every day. I had to alternate it. Some days I would do it and other days I wouldn't. I had to make sure I was drinking enough fluids on the fasting days because that would make it or break it. This plan also comes with some risks that you need to be aware of. One example is that it can lead to disordered eating, including binging, which is not good for anyone. It can cause a lot of health complications. Additionally, it can cause you to have fatigue, lightheadedness, constipation, and imbalances, making it very difficult for some people to deal with; therefore, you should do this type of fasting rarely, or only on special occasions.

Let me show you how I did a rigid three-week plan to get this thing started:

Week 1: "The Detox"

During this period, I drank vegetable juices, dairy products such as milk, cheese, and yogurt, and hard-boiled eggs for 20 hours per day. Once I got to the 4-hour eating period, I ate a large salad with a raspberry vinaigrette and lots of pinto beans, whole grain bread, plus some cheese and stir-fried vegetables. This created a balanced diet that did not involve binging or any other type of thing. There is a reason that this stage is called the "detoxing period," and it is a stage in which you don't want to do too much in the way of modifying your diet.

Week 2: Add Fat

During the second week, I would eat some apples and bananas, dairy products, hard-boiled eggs, and tomato juice for the first 20 hours. During the 4 hours, I would consume a massive salad with a balsamic vinaigrette and chicken breast, as well as stir-fried zucchini squash, plus some pinto beans. However, during this phase, I did not consume a lot of carbohydrates from whole grains or starches.

Week 3: Lose Fat

This third week was a time in which I loaded up on the carbs. On the first two days, I would eat foods high in carbs, then on days 3-4, I would eat foods that were high in protein, but low in carbs. Then, on days 5-6, I would eat foods that were high in carbs. Finally, on the last day or two, I would eat foods that would be high in protein, but low in carbs.

On the high-carb days, I would eat the same thing as before with 20 hours of eating vegetable juice, dairy products, hard-boiled eggs, and apples and bananas. During the 4 hour window, I would eat a large tuna salad with a vinaigrette and stir-fried vegetables, as well as one carb such as pasta, rice, or corn. On the low-carb days, I would eat the same thing as before with 20 hours of eating vegetable juice, dairy products, hard-boiled eggs, and dried fruits. During the 4 hour window, I would eat a salad with lots of raw veggies, plus a grilled chicken breast and some stir-fried zucchini. Finally, for dessert, I would have a mango smoothie.

My experience with this one was kind of hard. I tried it but, in the beginning, I would feel sluggish, and my energy level would be difficult to manage. I wanted to nap as soon as the day started and, also, working out was a nightmare the first week or so that I tried doing this. The first time I tried the warrior method, I was working out intensely, but my energy level was tanking as soon as I got back. Also, I was so freaking hungry that I wanted to gorge myself right after I hit the gym. I ended up drinking lots of coffee to fill up my energy reserves again. It was super difficult, and I started to lose motivation to work out anymore. As I went through it (it felt like hell for a few weeks), I was able to overcome the difficulty and gorge myself less. As soon as the 4 hour window started, I would stuff myself with steaks and pasta. Basically, I would eat the most unhealthy way possible. I would also eat a huge piece of cheesecake for dessert, and get a ton of fat into my system.

After a few weeks, I wanted to quit, and I got down on myself. I struggled with self-concept and wanted to give up, but then my trainer helped me to get my ass up and do some more lifting. I then managed and decided to do the Warrior Diet only every other week. It helped, and I saw some good positive results with my appetite and gained some muscle mass.

This type of workout is for the experts who have done the intermittent fasting routine for a while. I would not recommend it to beginners or intermediate-level fasters, because it requires discipline and withholding from going crazy during the overeating period of 4 hours. You may be tempted to eat whatever the heck you feel like during that time, and you might gorge yourself with fatty and high cholesterol foods. I don't think that gorging yourself is going to help out with weight loss or with adding muscle power to your routine.

It's hard to recommend this workout for people that want to have a healthy balance because it feels like you're doing a Thanksgiving-type feast every night, and I am sure that is not good. You might also not want to try eating a 3,000 calorie meal. That could be overkill. Be careful with this meal option and don't try it if you're just starting out. You should wait for a long time before you try it as an option because so many people do it the wrong way and they end up having a ton of problems. I don't want you to make costly mistakes that will destroy your motivation to continue. It is best to heed this caution. I'm warning you; this method is dangerous and to be used with the utmost care and discipline. I have tried to give you an example of how to responsibly handle those 4 hours for fasting. Follow the model with that type of food, and you will be in for a successful time.

Conclusion

To conclude this section, as you can see, there is a diet and meal plan for every stage of your journey with intermittent fasting. You can choose which plan to take, but I would urge you to begin with an 8-6 plan first, and then increase to a 16-8 plan because these plans can be easily built into your schedule and they don't cause too much disturbance in your daily living. While you may encounter some problems with them, you may be able to get used to it; however, it will take weeks, if not months or years to reap the benefits fully. Long-term weight loss will not happen unless you stick to it, so I would, therefore, advise you to stick to the plan religiously to get the best results. At the same time, you don't want to harm yourself in the process. If at any point you feel pain, you should stop fasting and eat something. Don't gorge yourself; give yourself a banana or a glass of warm milk.

Through each step of the process, you will notice how much easier it gets to do your fast. Your stomach will get used to it and allow you to feed on the right nutrients. Your body will store healthy fat in its system, to promote a good energy level to sustain you throughout your day. Also, be sure that you are staying hydrated all day long because there is nothing worse than going through a fast without drinking enough fluids - that means water, tea, coffee, Powerade/Gatorade, and fruit drinks.

Finally, I urge you to take action today. Your diet is going to be an essential part of helping you manage your weight, whether or not you choose to do intermittent fasting. You will need to make healthy decisions about what you will eat so that you don't overcompensate on the wrong things. I want you to be successful in this process. Take control of your diet and then choose a plan that will be best for you in the intermittent fasting process.

CHAPTER 8

(YEARS 5-6)

WORKOUT AND INTERMITTNET FASTING

In this chapter, I will show you how to develop a great body by forming a workout routine that will make you look like a hot dude or girl. This period was when I started integrating an organized workout routine into my plan, which was years 5-6. I will explain my story and then tell you how you can also accomplish this goal of having the body of your dreams.

As a young lad, I was really slim and skinny. You wouldn't believe how I looked before. I had a little bit of fat in my stomach from where I would not work out anything in my body. Honestly, I hated going to the gym. I didn't like other people watching me and looking at my body as I was running and struggling to work out on the treadmill or lift at the bench press. I was ashamed of my body and thought I would never measure up to other guys or their ability to lift over 200 pounds. As I went along with intermittent fasting in my fourth year, I realized that if I wanted to get healthier, I needed to buff up. So, in my fifth year, I hired a personal trainer who would help me to reach my goals of getting fitter. His name was Jamie, and he taught me a lot of things about how I could get better at my fitness.

Together, Jamie and I came up with a plan to increase my muscle mass. It was not easy at first because I had to focus on my diet and I had to add more protein and carbs to my diet to increase my weight. I had to add about 1,500 calories to my diet to do this, and it was not easy because I had to start eating once every 2 hours. Basically, I was scarfing down egg salad sandwiches and other things all day. I had to eat as much as possible to make sure that I wouldn't lose any weight.

The ways that we were going to increase my weight included going to the gym three times a week for weight training, and twice a week for endurance training. Three days a week - Monday, Wednesday, and Friday - I would go to the gym to do strength training to focus on building my biceps, triceps, and other muscles. In between those days, I would rest, and then I would do no work on the weekends. The key was to do short intensive strength training exercises. In between, I would relax my muscles and eat a lot. The key would become how I would eat and rest because those are the times that are the most extended. You have to take advantage of all that time that you're not working out and do your best to maintain that.

Exercising While Fasting

Exercising when fasting is an integral part of your wellness routine, but you have to watch out because it can come with risks. Some research has shown that exercising when you fast can cause insulin sensitivity and the control of blood sugar levels. This is important to keep in mind if you have diabetes, which I have. When you exercise while fasting, you will likely burn more fat that will make your workout harder, but you may also lose muscle mass while using up a lot of protein. That could deplete your system, and you will have less energy, so you have to be very careful.

When you're fasting, you will burn more fat, which will enable you to lose weight while burning more fat. You may also lose a lot of energy by working this way, and you might not perform at your best. Also, you might lose muscle mass in the process, which will hinder your ability to build the muscle that you want.

The Solution to Dealing with the Challenges

When you're planning to work out while fasting, there are some considerations you should make. First, you should think about exactly when you will do the workout. One popular method is to use the 16-8 window, wherein you will do all your eating within 8 hours and fast for 16 hours. For better performance, it is best to plan your workouts within this 8 hour window, because then you will have the fuel that will keep you going for a length of time.

Secondly, you should choose a suitable type of workout based on the timing of your meals. You want to have a higher carb diet on days that you do your strength training, but you could do an endurance training day on days with low carbs.

Thirdly, if you work out, you need to plan on replenishing your body with energy and protein immediately upon completing your workout.

The main things to keep in mind is that you need to eat close to the time when you are doing your high-intensity workouts, and you need to drink lots of water and energy drinks to keep your body going through all aspects of the training. You should drink Gatorade or Powerade to have a higher electrolytes level. Also, with the intensity of the workout, you should keep it short and simple to avoid strain or injury that could come from working out too hard.

Finally, you need to listen to your body. If you feel hungry, eat. Don't allow your body to go for too long without food. When you exercise while fasting, undoubtedly, you will become hungrier with each passing minute. It is crucial that you get all the intake of calories and carbs in as soon as this happens because you will need to replenish the protein that is lost during intensive workouts. Also, make sure to include periods of rest in your routine that will enable you to do recover from intense workout cycles that can cause trauma to your system.

My Example

As I began my workout, I decided that I wanted to gain muscle mass. I was unsure how to go about it because I hadn't worked on it before. My personal trainer put me on a workout plan, and he worked with me on how to gain muscle mass, and we co-ordinated my meals around my workout times. I would work out in the afternoon just right before dinner so that I would be able to eat a high carb and protein meal with over 2,000 calories right away. That would immediately replenish all the protein I had lost during the workout, and then, I would eat less the next day in between workouts. I would always eat, work out, replenish and do this continuously to get the results that I desired. It worked for me.

Within a few months, I was able to build muscle mass. I gained 10lbs and could see the results in my biceps as I could see that there was some definition that was developing there. I was satisfied and thanked my personal trainer for helping me.

How It Can Help You Lose Weight

Because you may be eating during the cycles that you work out, you will lose some weight in the process while burning fat. It may be hard to do at first, but you have to time it just right. If your goal is to lose fat, then a good way is to time your workouts around the time of your fast but, then again, you might lose muscle mass, so be careful. Likewise, it is a good idea to do your workout during your time of eating, because your metabolism will get a boost of energy and you will see that you want more food; therefore, you will burn more calories and get a good result.

Conclusion

To sum up, working out while fasting is a great idea and can come with many benefits, but you also have to watch out and make sure you're not overdoing it. Also, you have to time your workouts at the right time and to replenish the energy that you will lose while working out. You don't want to get light-headed, dizzy, or have a headache from overdoing working out on an empty stomach. It is never a good idea. Be sure to take good care of yourself at all times so that you don't cause this problem. It is never a good idea to overdo the workout just so that you can lose a couple of pounds. You will develop a lot more risks and, potentially experience hazards that could be very dangerous for your health.

Once you decide on a good workout plan with a personal trainer or a trusted friend, you will be able to develop a useful framework for working out safely and effectively. Develop a game plan and stick to it, along with a diet that will work wonders for your overall health. Finally, have confidence that you are meant to achieve your dreams and goals in your health. All things are possible when you can carefully plan your future with achievable goals, so believe that it is possible. I know you can do it.

CHAPTER 9

(YEARS 7-10)

BENEFITS I AM SEEING IN MY BODY

In this chapter, I am going to highlight to you how I saw benefits in my body, work, relationships, and family. Intermittent fasting made a massive difference in my life, and I want to share with you how it all came about.

Before I started on this journey, I suffered from acid reflux, which also caused me to have "freaking heartburn." It happened after eating spicy food, but it also happened when I ate anything with fat or protein. My esophagus would burn like Hades, and I would have to go to the bathroom many times a day. It was so miserable. I went to the doctor and had to take heartburn pills for my acid reflux. One time I even had to go to the emergency room for having heart palpitations after eating a spicy Korean kimchi soup. It was horrible. I got out soon after that, but it was also at that point that I realized that I needed to take control of my health and what I ate. I would sometimes feel a terrible aching stomach pain that wouldn't go away unless I took medication for the condition. Day in, day out, I was going to the doctor for heartburn pain and feeling freaking miserable all the time. It was so hard, and I knew that I needed to get some help for it. The bloating and gas problem was a continual problem that I struggled with before doing intermittent fasting, as well.

After I decided to undertake the intermittent fasting in my third year, I started to notice the difference with my body. It took a while to get to this point, but I no longer felt like I had a bloating sensation. I no longer had a heaviness in my stomach every time I would eat something spicy. I was able to enjoy all the Korean and Indian food that my heart desired because I was able to take care of myself. I didn't have as much gas and the tendency to let it out at times, which was good, because my farts stank so much afterwards. It had to do with what I was eating, but also was due to the heartburn problem. I felt and looked better. No more of that sour feeling in my esophagus as soon as I downed a spicy chilly pepper from the Mexican restaurant. I felt loads better in what I could eat. I also was able to go to the bathroom easier. It made a big difference.

With my body, I could see and feel a tangible difference. I looked and felt great. I had a lot more energy from intermittent fasting and workouts. I was able to get the rest that I needed every night, and slept better as a result. Consequently, I got up every morning with a new sense of energy and determination to "seize the day." I was so excited to go to work and complete the projects that I had. Into my fifth year in the program, I enrolled in a financial advisor course at the local university. Within six months, I got my financial advisor license. I started working at an office in the downtown area and was making more money. I started making 50K per year and gradually increased my salary above that. I eventually was able to move out of my parents' house and rent my own place in the center of downtown LA. I bought a Ferrari and was able to score the job of my dreams. After I turned 34, I was really living it up and feeling prosperous as a young, single male. I enjoyed my singleness as a great time in my life.

I credit all this goal achievement to my discipline in doing this fasting routine. It made a huge difference. I knew that I needed to do all these things because I believed in myself. I also wanted to set high goals and objectives for myself because I knew I could accomplish more. My self-esteem increased over time, and then I knew that I could do all the things that I set my mind to because I had the discipline and willpower to get it done.

Additionally, my relationship with my parents improved. I enjoyed going home and talking to my mom and dad. I had a more positive attitude while talking to them and enjoyed helping them around the house. They were also more accommodating and welcoming to my new intermittent and workout schedule. Mom, especially, was happy to see that I had a healthy appetite. When I was younger, I used to be a very picky eater. I didn't enjoy eating fruit and vegetables, and my parents are vegan, so it helped that we were able to tackle this problem through the intermittent fasting. My parents saw me eating more healthily, and they wanted to help me with buying my food. They even got some fresh ingredients for me to cook at home. Mom let me help her with the gardening, and we grew some fresh tomatoes.

When I turned 35, I finally decided that I wanted to start dating. I was a shy guy and didn't want to be in a relationship. I was too self-conscious of my lean body and didn't want to have a girlfriend. As soon as I started working out and building muscle mass, I noticed that my testosterone level started going up and I became more interested in women, and then I realized that I wanted to date a woman. I started picking up women and dated several girls. It was hard at first, and I got my heart broken a couple of times but, when I reached age 36, I found the girl of my dreams. Her name was Rachel, and she was terrific. We immediately understood each other. She was attracted to me because I was a goal-oriented and hardworking man. We went out for a few months and, in the summer of that year, I got engaged to her. It was awesome.

As you can see, this intermittent fasting routine helped me so much, and I got to meet different people and finally met my wife-to-be. After doing the method for a while, I got out of my singleness and aspired for more. I wanted to become a husband. It changed my life priorities, and I realized that I had to aspire to be great and to achieve what had been seemingly impossible before.

What All This Means for You

If you're reading this, then you know that you have to take action. You can't just sit on your ass and do nothing about it. You have to get out there and do it. You've got to get out there and do your thing, and that means that you can also get the body that you desire with the muscle mass that you want. You are going to have to set goals for yourself and schedule the time to do all the things you need to do. Schedule your fast, watch your diet and you will be able to accomplish your goal. You should also put that picture of yourself, that you want to be, on your mirror. Maybe that's a Hugh Jackman or Tom Cruise picture. Imagine yourself with that six pack and huge biceps, and then, get 'er done. Go to the gym. Go swimming. Lift weights. Do all that is necessary to build up your physique. Eat like crazy for 8 hours during your day - once every hour or two. Snacking also helps you. Engage in your physical exercise.

If you follow through with all the things above, then you can start building muscle mass, and then fast and rest. Enjoy the time when you're not eating or doing activities. Rest is so crucial to your wellbeing. Believe that you can do it. It won't be easy. You might be tired and frustrated a lot of the time. I know I felt like shit sometimes and wanted to quit. I got so tired of not eating and was so tempted to break the fast and eat a bag of Cheetos while watching Grey's Anatomy re-runs. Believe me, I've been there. It felt like rock bottom and was freaking depressing. What I am saying is that it is worth all of it, because you can go for that goal with all your might and achieve the body of your dreams, because you have envisioned it in your heart.

Conclusion

To conclude, I think that it is essential to keep in mind continually your goal and the body you want to get. Having a mental picture of the man that you want to be is important because you have to strive and do your best to achieve it. Don't think for a second that it won't involve you stretching yourself, because if you think it's a smooth ride and you can sit on your ass and vedge on Netflix every day, then you're in for a hard time. I'm not going to lie to you. It's going to suck sometimes. You're going to want to cry and sulk when you can't reach for that gallon of ice cream after 6pm and eat your feelings. You're going to ache and groan from the pain of not taking in any calories. You might have a headache. Heck, you might fall flat on your face because you haven't eaten in 15 hours. I've been there. I know the pain. It sucks but, once you've reached your breaking point, you will realize how strong of a man you are. You know that you have overcome so much in your life. This was one small inkling of a time when you had to endure and, no matter how painful as shit this time is, you know that you will be able to achieve your dream and that makes you want to celebrate your achievement. Do it because you care about yourself. Do it because you want to be a better man. Do it so that you can get the ladies to come and go out with you.

I was successful with it, and I know that you can be, too. Hang in there friend, I know you can do it. It's going to be hard, but once you've accomplished it, there will be a wave of euphoria that will change your life. This is going to be a long road to the finish line. It took me ten years to get where I am, but every step of the way made a difference and I am a better man as a result. I believe you can do it too, so let's do this thing!

CHAPTER 10

THE MAN I AM TODAY (10 YEARS LATER)

Here I am. It is my 38th birthday, and I am 10 years into this intermittent fasting journey. There's been a lot of heartache through these years. I now want to tell you where I am at after these ten years and what my dreams and hopes are for the future, as well as pointers for you to have.

I've already told you about how I started this journey with no ambition and only wanted to get by and pay my bills and live in my parents' basement. Since starting the journey, I moved out of my parents' house, got my own place and lived alone for a while, got an fantastic job and a great car and house, and then got married. All these things happened over time as I wanted to achieve each milestone. Not bad for a man who had no ambition, right?

The point I have wanted to get across to you in this book is that you have to have some ambition to get where you want to be. You must set a target and goal for yourself. I was able to do that every step of the way while approaching each part of the journey with care and dedication. It was a lot of hard work and blood, sweat, and tears. There were moments where I sat on the toilet and was crapping a boatload because I had an upset stomach from working out too much and not eating enough. Those headaches would hurt like shit, and I found myself dazed and confused at times. Sometimes, I struggled with insomnia because of hunger pains. As we saw before, I had a series of struggles and mistakes that I made that were difficult for me. At the end of the ten years, I made it through. I went through all the meal plans that I have described in detail. I did the 8-6, 16-8, the 5-2, and the warrior plan for several years, alternating between plans each month and year.

I will be honest with you. I struggled a lot with motivation on my own. I needed accountability. That's why I talked to my trusted friend and trainer Jamie. We worked together throughout those years, and Jamie became like a best friend to me. We enjoyed hanging out together frequently, and we eventually got to go traveling together to Europe and Asia. I opened up to Jamie about my struggles. I would highly recommend that you also find a trusted friend to reach out to in this process. There's no way to go on this journey alone; you need to have accountability. Trust me on this point.

In all my time, I have needed not only the support of my trusted friend and trainer, but also my friends and family. Over time, people became kinder and supportive of the kind of efforts I was making. People no longer made fun of me. They saw the difference to my body that this fasting was making. They saw the six-pack and muscle definition that I was getting over time. Men and women were admiring my body, and I knew that it was making a difference. People became attracted to me and my positivity. I was glowing with pride every time I'd talk about intermittent fasting and how it had changed my life. They also felt like they could relate to my story because it is relevant and makes people think about their own lives. I knew that this journey had started and ended with some good fodder to help others get started with their journey.

So, I have to ask you, are you ready to begin? I want you to be prepared for a transformation, and I want to give you all the tools and tips that will help you successfully launch your intermittent fasting training plan. You've seen what a difference it has made in my life. I believe it can also happen in your life. I am excited to share some of the powerful tips that you can use to begin the adventure of your life. It's not only going to be for a year or two; it's going to be the adventure of a lifetime. You will make decisions and cultivate habits that will follow you for the rest of your life. I know, because I am going to use the habits I have formed through this process for a very long time. It's ingrained into who I am.

Let's do this thing. Read on to find out about the tips that will help you to get started in the next and final chapter of the book.

CHAPTER 11

POWERFUL TIPS TO MAKE YOU START NOW

As you have seen so far in this book, intermittent fasting changed my life. It has a host of benefits that have made me more confident in myself and have led me to pursue a life of greatness, which is following my heart's desire to get lean and fit. Over the past ten years, many people have wanted to know more about intermittent fasting and its popularity. Intermittent fasting has many benefits that include weight loss, reversing type 2 diabetes, savings in time and money, among others.

In this chapter, we are going to show you how you can get the most out of your fasting routine. Let's begin with the basics:

How Long Do You Want to Fast?

24-hour Fasts

This is a way of fasting from dinner to dinner (or lunch to lunch). For example, if you eat dinner on the first day, you would not eat breakfast the next day or lunch and then eat dinner again the following day. In this case, you would be eating once daily. It would be recommended that you do this type of fast only two to three times per week. You can get the most benefits by doing this because you can replenish your energy one time per day and then fast for 24 hours. This is an effective means to do it.

My Example

I usually do this type of fasting once or twice a week. It has helped me to maintain my metabolism and restores my system after eating many heavy meals. It has helped me to keep a healthy weight and has given me some flexibility in varying my time spent in fasting.

5:2 Fast

This fast is done when you have five days where you eat regularly and two fasting days; however, on the fast days, you take in only 500 calories each day. You can consume these calories either all at once or spread out throughout the day.

My Example

Every two weeks, I do this type of fasting, and it helps me when I feel weak and need time to recharge my system. I have found that if I can take it easy on the fasting for a few days in a month, it helps me to do better, and I also don't have as many hunger pains in my system and a stomach ache that hurts terribly.

36-hour Fasts

During this fast, you would fast for the entire day. You would eat dinner on the first day, and then fast for the whole day of the second day, and then not eat again until day three at breakfast time. This type of fasting is used to promote weight loss. Also, it allows you not to be tempted to overeat on the second day.

My Example

I do this fast once a month, like when I want to do a spiritual retreat and meditate. I go up to a mountain and don't eat and spend some time reflecting and meditating. It is excellent, and I can truly connect with my feelings and emotions.

Shorter Fasts

Many people will do a 16-8 fast. In this fast, you do it for 16 hours, and then you eat within a window of 8 hours. During the eight hours, you consume all the nutrients in your system. To be honest, this is the fast that I do most of the time. It is something that Hugh Jackman once recommended, and I want to recommend it to you. For most people, this type of fast is totally possible and doesn't require much thought or effort on the part of the person fasting.

Within the eight hours, a person does not eat anything, and then a person will eat all his or her meals between 11:00 am and 7:00 pm. Many people choose to skip breakfast during this time, but others skip dinner and only eat breakfast and lunch.

In my case, I decided I wanted to do intermittent fasting by skipping breakfast. Instead of eating anything for breakfast, I decided to opt for something that many people in America want - coffee. It gets me through the day and allows me to wake up without having to overeat in the morning. And then I eat lunch and dinner. It saves me a heck of a lot of money, time, and energy to prepare breakfast, and I'd recommend that you try it as well.

There is also the 20-4 fast. During this time, you eat during a 4-hour eating window and then fast for 20 hours. I found that this method was not as effective, and I would often have a terrible headache by fasting for about twenty hours. I wouldn't recommend this one, as it did cause me a lot of problems.

What are Some of the Side Effects that I Might Encounter?

As with any diet plan, there are risks to consider, and you should consult a doctor or a trusted person who can guide you through this process. I am no doctor, so don't quote me on this information, but I think that it is crucial that you find a way of working with a professional, who can aid in different dietary and medical needs that you may have. If you are taking medication, I would strongly advise consulting a doctor, because who knows what might happen if you start fasting and then you have high blood pressure or some other result. You want to be careful.

Hunger: You will likely experience severe pain whenever you fast, and you might get a rumbling of your stomach during lunch, which may continue for a long time. Those hunger groans may happen for a while, so you have to be careful. You may also have a stomach ache after not eating for a while.

Headaches: You may experience migraines or other problems that can be painful to endure. It will be hard on your system, and you might seriously want to quit the program at this point, but I would advise you to stick through it.

Constipation: Because you're not eating as much, you won't have to go to the bathroom as much, and it may make you less regular to go to the toilet. Try a laxative if you cannot go to the bathroom for an extended period.

Hazy feeling and lightheadedness: Whenever you do your intermittent fasting plus exercise, you will feel a bit light-headed so prepare for this, especially in the beginning. You're going to struggle with doing your day-to-day activities because it is brand new to you.

Low energy, especially in the beginning: When you start exercising and fasting, you will lose a lot of energy first, because your body is getting used to fasting and exercising. Be ready to handle this aspect.

Lack of motivation and a desire to quit: This is the one that we all will encounter at some point in our lives. There is a genuine desire to quit that you may experience when you're on this journey that you're going to have to be ready for. It will hit you like a red brick sometimes, so you're going to have to brace yourself for it before it affects you. While it is challenging at the start, it will get better with time.

Desire to binge when eating and do unhealthy things: One last point is that you want to avoid binging on foods, but it will be a temptation that you will inevitably have. When a person is hungry, he will want to vedge out, so you will have to learn how to deal with this side effect.

What Are Some of the Things to Keep in Mind During a Fast?

Stay hydrated. Drink lots of water during your intermittent fasting. I cannot stress this point enough. You have to drink as much water as possible because you have to take care of yourself. Your body is made up of mostly water, so you have to make sure you're getting enough water in your system daily. Don't ever skimp on this point. You can also be hydrated by ways other than just water;

for example, you could drink energy drinks or other things like that. The important thing is not to do too much activity without water or other beverages. This is especially the case if you are exercising or working out a lot.

Keep a busy schedule. Another thing you have to do is stay busy because this will make a difference in how you can live a good life. There is an old saying that says "Idleness is a devil's tool." I think that is true. You have to stay busy to get ahead in life. You cannot just sit on your ass all day, watch TV re-runs, and do other things. You have to do a lot of things in your life. Enjoy socializing with others. Have a life. Get ahead in your career. There are a lot of things that I would recommend you to do. You have to make the most of every moment, because the thing is, this life is short. You've got to get a lot out of it and make a meaningful life, and that does not mean sitting around and doing nothing and waiting for someone to tell you what to do. It means having a game plan and sticking to it. This will help you to enjoy your fasting more. You will not even notice that you took the time out of your schedule to fast because you will be so busy doing all the things that make a difference in the world.

Have a cup of coffee or tea. This point is so important. Tea and coffee are filled with antioxidants and are useful to help you have more energy, and we know that caffeine is what keeps most of the world going. Coffee also has a natural appetite suppressant that enables you to go for longer without eating anything.

Keep trying, don't give up. I would also recommend that you keep trying and do not give up because the plan should be in place, such that you will achieve your goal, whether that is weight loss or some other plan, so keep doing it. You can do it! I believe you can. Trust me. It's hard, and it will take some hard work, but it is worth everything for you to achieve that body that you deserve to have.

Don't eat too much after fasting. One thing that you definitely should avoid is binging after you fast. If you do a fast, you should avoid having a feast the day you stop. Not a good idea, believe me, been there, done that. I vomited up a storm after it. Horrible. Never again. I would highly recommend that you do not overeat. Don't go out to Cracker Barrel or the Golden Corral following an extended period of fasting.

Break the fast gradually. This point goes with #5. You have to be gradual with resuming your regular dieting. It is crucial that you return with a little bit at a time, rather than overloading your system, which can lead to complications and difficulties. You don't want to shock your system with food and cause stomach pain or other abdominal conditions.

Who Shouldn't Fast?

Another point we need to go over is who are the people who shouldn't fast. First, if you are underweight and have a low BMI, it is highly recommended that you don't fast. Also, pregnant women should not try intermittent fasting. Finally, people that are involved in intensely athletic activities, such as team sports, should take care not to fast because of the high energy that is exerted within those activities.

How to Begin Now

Ok, so now you have decided to do intermittent fasting. Congratulations! You're ready to embark on this fantastic adventure that you will not regret that you did. I know that you have looked at many case studies in this book of how I was able to use intermittent fasting and it changed my life. I am no longer the same man. I think that you can also do the same thing. So, if you're committed to seeing your life change, let's begin now. Here are the action steps that I would recommend you take in the coming days:

Decide on what type of fast you want to do. Is the 16-8 fast ideal for your schedule? What about the 5-2 fast? The 24-hour fast? Think about which option you want to do. You should carefully consider which one fits your needs, body type, and goal, etc.

Decide how long it will be for. Will this fast be for one week, two weeks, or longer? Choose a duration for your program, and how long you will do it. Often, our bodies are created to do some activity for a period of time, but in brief spurts. Think of when you were studying 8 hours a day for final exams when you were in college. The same principle applies here, so choose a duration that is appropriate for your project.

Start fasting! Now that you have planned your fast, do it! You can do it! It will be amazing. It will be tough, and you may want to quit, but you have to carry out your project and do it with passion.

Continue doing your everyday activities as usual. Even when you're fasting, you can continue doing your day-to-day activities as you did before. It will take time to get used to it; however, you will need to make your system adjust.

Break the fast at an appropriate time. After this, you should break your fast gradually, and without binging or having a feast so that you won't get sick.

Repeat your fast within a designated period.

Conclusion

Now that you have an excellent resource from my experience and knowledge, you can use it to start your own intermittent fasting plan. Follow the steps and method that I have outlined for you with the tips, and you will be able to see the results you want to see. The main thing you need to do is have a game plan that you can stick to. It needs to have a clear and achievable goal that you can use. Choose your fast, the duration, and how you will do it. Schedule your meals. Keep in mind the precautions and warnings that we have highlighted here. Be careful and take the right measures to protect your health. If you feel unbearable pain, you should stop fasting and eat something right away. We don't want you to do something dangerous to your health. Take good care of yourself. You can and will succeed if you follow our detailed instructions, and I am a living testimonial to how it has worked for me.

CONCLUSION OF CHAPTERS

To wrap up what we have talked about, I want to inspire you to think big about your life. We only live maybe 70 or 80 years at most on average, and we have to get the most out of our lives. I want you to live an amazing life that is filled with joy, peace, and prosperity. I don't want you to waste your time trying to figure out a strategy that may or may not work from a fancy expensive diet plan. What I have offered you is a simple solution that has positive and significant results with intermittent fasting.

I was a shy, lanky man before, who had no kind of physique before starting a diet and intermittent fasting plan. As I said in the introduction, I had no plan for my life, no way going forward because I was so focused on fleeting pleasures. I was going to lose out on so many things because I was not paying attention to my health. Learning about my diabetes diagnosis and my mom's death from cancer, I felt that I needed to take the necessary steps to protect my health, because, the truth is, it's a gift to have good health. No-one is entitled to it. If you're lucky enough to not get sick in a year, then you are living a good life.

Don't you want to live a life filled with good health? Don't you want to have a hot body that everyone wants? Do you want to have a girlfriend or boyfriend that you know you deserve? Look no further than intermittent fasting. It is a proven technique that works. Many celebrities, including Hugh Jackman, have endorsed it and use it regularly. If you can make intermittent fasting part of your diet routine, you may see some sustained and extensive results to your weight management plan, and you may be able to lose the weight that you have now.

Don't think for a moment that it is going to be easy. I have already enumerated the struggles, pain, and anxiety that I had to go through to get where I am now. It took a lot of difficulty and challenges to arrive at the point where I am today. I couldn't get through it without the support of my parents, friends, trainer, and my wife. All my loved ones eventually jumped on the bandwagon and supported me in all the efforts that I made. That has made the most significant difference in my life; therefore, I urge you to get the kind of support system that is going to allow you to achieve the results that you desire. It's going to be hard to do it on your own; I would say, impossible. No person can operate on their own. Everyone needs someone else to help them. We're meant to live our lives in community with one another. That means supporting the weaker person and encouraging them. You need someone to cheer you on the race to the finish line. Life is a marathon; you've got to pace yourself and have your cheerleaders to back you up when the going gets tough.

As you go through this journey, I recommend you look back at this small book of tips, experience, and ideas for inspiration. Remember the struggles that I have highlighted to you. Recall the adventure that it was for me. There were some fantastic victories that I experienced, and I was so glad to reach different milestones throughout my life. I believe that with patience, hard work, endurance, and perseverance, it is absolutely possible for you to achieve the milestones that you have set for yourself in your own life.

Here is my last call to action. Get out there. Do your thing. Start exercising. Go to the gym and get on an exercise plan. Run laps, swim in the pool, do whatever floats your boat and find some muscle exercises that will strengthen your core. Choose a workout plan and meal plan that will enable you to do the fasts that you want to do to get the results. Stick to your project like a religion. You have to be consistent if you're going to see the results that you want. Hang in there when the going gets tough; it won't always be easy. You may be excited at the beginning of the journey, but that excitement will wane over time. You still have to keep going. Keep your eye on the prize - whether that is to lose weight, gain muscle mass, or just live a healthy lifestyle.

Made in United States
North Haven, CT
20 June 2023

38029715R00059